Unlocking the Hidden Pillars of Intimacy

A Comprehensive Guide to Building Deep Emotional Bonds, Nurturing Authentic Relationships, and Cultivating Lasting Fulfillment in Love, Life, and Beyond

Cheryl Bach

Unlocking the Hidden Pillars of Intimacy

Cheryl Bach

Table of Contents

Unlocking the Hidden Pillars of Intimacy

Chapter I.

Introduction

A. Overview of the Importance of Intimacy

Intimacy is a fundamental part of human nature that can form the foundation of deep emotional bonds and authentic relationships. It is an intricate yet important aspect of life that plays a vital role in cultivating lasting fulfillment in love, life, and beyond. Despite its significance, many people find intimacy to be a complex and challenging terrain.

The term intimacy refers to a variety of experiences, including emotional, intellectual, spiritual, and physical. Intimacy creates a space for individuals to connect, share and communicate with one another freely. It is a nurturing and supportive tool that helps create strong connections

Unlocking the Hidden Pillars of Intimacy

among humans with different personalities and is necessary for growth and nurture of healthy relationships.

B. Purpose of the Book

The purpose of this book is to serve as a comprehensive guide to unlocking the hidden pillars of intimacy. The book aims to provide you with an in-depth understanding of the nature of intimacy, the importance of building deep emotional bonds and nurturing authentic relationships, and how cultivating intimacy can lead to lasting fulfillment in love, life, and beyond.

This book is intended for those who are seeking to enhance their understanding of intimacy, and those who are trying to create more authentic and deeper connections with others. It is also useful for people who are looking to heal past wounds or build stronger relationships with a partner or family member.

Cheryl Bach

C. Outline of the Book

The book is divided into four sections, each focusing on a different aspect of intimacy:

Section 1: Foundations of Intimacy

This section provides the foundational knowledge needed to understand intimacy, including a definition of intimacy, the different types of intimacy, and the role that relationships play in facilitating intimacy.

Section 2: Developing Emotional Bonds

In this section, the book explores how to create emotional bonds with others, including understanding your own emotions, connecting with others in meaningful ways, and incorporating vulnerability into relationships.

Section 3: Nurturing Authentic Relationships

The third section focuses on building authentic relationships with others by exploring communication skills, effective conflict resolution, and establishing trust, respect, and healthy boundaries.

Section 4: Cultivating Lasting Fulfillment

Finally, this section covers practices for cultivating lasting fulfillment in life, love, and beyond, including self-care, self-awareness, and exploring spiritual and personal growth.

Through the pages of this book, you will be able to harness the power of intimacy and use it as a tool to build deeper, more meaningful connections with others. They will gain insight into their own emotions, develop the skills needed for effective communication and conflict resolution, and learn how to establish trust, respect, and boundaries in all of their relationships.

Cheryl Bach

In summary, this book is designed to provide a comprehensive guide to unlocking the hidden pillars of intimacy. With it, you can begin to explore new depths of emotional connection in all aspects of their lives, creating a richer, more fulfilling experience of love, life, and beyond.

Chapter II.

Foundations of Intimacy

A. Understanding Intimacy

Intimacy is a complex and multifaceted experience that is essential in building deep emotional bonds, nurturing authentic relationships, and cultivating lasting fulfillment in love, life, and beyond. At its core, intimacy is about building connection and creating an environment where two individuals can share their thoughts, feelings, and desires with each other in a safe, respectful, and meaningful way.

Intimacy can come in various forms, ranging from emotional, intellectual, spiritual, and of course, physical. Each form of intimacy plays an important role in creating a well-rounded, fulfilling relationship. Furthermore, intimacy is a dynamic process that evolves over time, requiring both partners to actively work on it in order to maintain a healthy and fulfilling relationship.

B. Discovering Your Personal Needs and Values

In order to build intimacy with another person, it's important to first understand and acknowledge your own needs and values. This means taking the time to reflect on what you truly want and need in a relationship, as well as what your core values and beliefs are. Without this understanding, it can be difficult to establish a deep and meaningful connection with someone else.

One way to discover your personal needs and values is through self-reflection and introspection. Start by asking yourself questions such as: What do I want in a relationship? What are my deal-breakers? What are my values and beliefs? Taking the time to explore these questions can help you become more aware of yourself and your desires, making it easier to communicate them with your partner.

C. Creating Safe Space for Emotional Expression

Creating a safe space for emotional expression is crucial in building intimacy and deepening emotional bonds with your partner. In order to do this, it's important that both partners feel comfortable expressing their emotions without fear of judgement or rejection.

One way to create a safe space for emotional expression is by actively listening to your partner. This means giving them your undivided attention, asking open-ended questions, and showing empathy and understanding towards their emotions. It's also important to avoid interrupting, criticizing, or dismissing your partner's emotions, as this can make them feel invalidated and unheard.

Unlocking the Hidden Pillars of Intimacy

Another way to create a safe space for emotional expression is by setting boundaries and respecting each other's limits. This means being willing to compromise and communicate effectively when conflicts arise, and understanding that healthy relationships require mutual respect and trust between partners.

By cultivating a safespace for emotional expression, both partners can begin to share their thoughts and feelings more freely, which in turn can lead to a deeper and more meaningful connection. This connection can help to fulfill some of the core needs that we have as human beings, such as love, belonging, and validation.

In summary, developing intimacy requires an understanding of what intimacy is, discovering your personal needs and values, and creating a safe space for emotional expression. By actively working on these foundational pillars of intimacy, you can build a deeper, more fulfilling relationship with your partner.

Chapter III.

Building Deep Emotional Bonds

A. Unveiling Vulnerability and Authenticity

In today's society, vulnerability is often seen as a weakness. However, in building deep emotional bonds, vulnerability is one of the key ingredients to fostering intimacy. Unveiling vulnerability requires the courage to share our thoughts, feelings, and experiences with another person without fear of rejection or judgement.

To cultivate vulnerability and authenticity in a relationship, it's essential to create a safe space for open communication. This involves active listening, placing value on your partner's perspective, and responding to their emotions with empathy and understanding. True authenticity can be achieved if both partners feel comfortable being their true selves in the relationship while expressing themselves freely.

B. Enhancing Trust and Commitment

Trust and commitment are critical components of building deep emotional bonds. Trust is built over time, and it grows as individuals demonstrate reliability, consistency, honesty, and integrity in their words and actions towards each other.

To enhance trust, it's essential to communicate openly and honestly, keep promises, and follow through on commitments. Regularly checking in with one another and giving affirmations and reassurance can also show your commitment to building a strong bond.

Commitment is more than just the words you say or the promises you make; it's also about investing energy, effort, and resources into the relationship. This means taking the time to prioritize the relationship and make it a focal point of your life. By making this investment, partners can foster a deeper sense of connection and trust with each other.

C. Communicating Effectively in Relationships

Effective communication is the backbone of all healthy relationships. To communicate effectively, partners need to be mindful of their words, tone, and timing. It's essential to listen actively, seek to understand each other's perspectives, and respond honestly.

One way to improve communication is to set aside dedicated time for authentic conversations. These conversations can allow partners to speak openly and honestly about their needs, desires, fears, and concerns. It's also important to communicate regularly, not just when something needs to be discussed or resolved.

Non-verbal communication can also play a significant role in building deep emotional bonds. This can include eye contact, facial expressions, touch, and body language. Being attuned to these subtle cues can enhance understanding and reinforce emotional connection.

To summarize, building deep emotional bonds requires vulnerability, trust, commitment, and effective communication. Creating a safe, supportive space for open, authentic conversations, prioritizing the relationship, and being mindful of non-verbal communication can help partners build a more profound, intimate connection. It takes effort and patience to build deep emotional bonds, but the rewards are a relationship strengthened by mutual love, support, and understanding. Finally, while building connections with others can be challenging, it's essential to remember that both partners should share the responsibility of creating deeper intimacy in their relationship. By consistently working towards building deep emotional bonds, couples can cultivate lasting fulfillment in life.

Chapter IV.

Nurturing Authentic Relationships

A. Differentiating Love and Romance

At times, people often confuse love and romance, and that can be detrimental to nurturing authentic relationships. Romance involves the expression of intense attraction or infatuation, while love is a deeper and more sustained emotional connection with someone.

It's important to communicate honestly what love means to us, what we want from a relationship, and our expectations. Being clear about our definition of love can help us recognize the difference between fleeting romance and long-lasting emotional bonds. Remember, love is built on communication, respect, trust, and support, not just physical appearances and grand gestures.

B. Cultivating Intentional Connections

Authentic relationships require intentional connections, meaning taking the time and effort to nurture the relationship actively. This includes prioritizing the relationship above other distractions, such as work or hobbies, and making time for meaningful shared experiences.

It's also essential to be present in the moment when spending time with a partner. This means putting away distractions like your phone or work-related emails and fully engaging with your partner. Focusing on strengthening your connection through shared activities, exploring new interests together, and investing time and energy into building the relationship can go a long way towards nurturing an authentic bond.

C. Practicing Forgiveness and Gratitude

Inevitably, all relationships face challenges, disagreements, and mistakes. Practicing forgiveness is crucial for building and maintaining an authentic relationship. When conflicts arise, it's important to actively listen to the other person's perspective and acknowledge if mistakes were made. However, moving forward requires letting go of resentment and forgiving one another.

On the flip side, feelings of gratitude can strengthen authentic connections. Practicing gratitude involves recognizing the things we appreciate about our partner, celebrating their accomplishments, and expressing our appreciation through actions or words. This practice can create a positive feedback loop; feeling appreciated can boost our relationship satisfaction, leading us to be more grateful and intentional with our partner in return.

By practicing forgiveness and gratitude, couples can create a foundation of mutual understanding, respect, and acceptance. Addressing conflict with openness and compassion allows relationships to grow and evolve without being bogged down by resentment and grudges.

In conclusion, nurturing authentic relationships requires intentionality, communication, forgiveness, and gratitude. By prioritizing shared experiences, being present in the moment, and recognizing the difference between love and romance, couples can build deep emotional bonds that last. Conflict is inevitable, but by actively seeking forgiveness and expressing gratitude, couples can overcome obstacles and strengthen their relationships in the long term. When couples work together to nurture their relationships, they create a safe and supportive space for love, growth, and fulfillment.

Unlocking the Hidden Pillars of Intimacy

To reinforce the importance of nurturing authentic relationships, it's essential to recognize how they contribute to our overall sense of wellbeing. People who have strong emotional bonds with their partners tend to report higher levels of life satisfaction, better mental health, and even improved physical health. This is because emotional intimacy provides us with a sense of security, validation, and companionship.

In contrast, struggling relationships can lead to feelings of loneliness, rejection, and even depression. While every relationship will face challenges, neglecting to address issues or failing to intentionally nurture the relationship can lead to prolonged unhappiness and despair.

Ultimately, nurturing authentic relationships means putting in the time, effort, and dedication needed to create a deep and lasting connection with your partner. By focusing on communication, mutual understanding, and emotional intimacy, couples can build trust, support, and fulfillment into their daily lives. As with any aspect of life, what we put out into our relationships is what we'll get back. So invest in your relationship and watch it bloom into something beautiful and lasting.

To start building authentic connections, prioritize communication, set aside quality time together, and express forgiveness and gratitude. Through these practices, you can create a relationship that fosters emotional growth, exploration, and eventual fulfillment.

By differentiating love and romance, cultivating intentional connections, and practicing forgiveness and gratitude, couples can unlock the hidden pillars of intimacy and create something truly special. So go ahead and invest in your relationship, make the effort to nurture and foster your bond, and reap the rewards of authentic love and happiness that are waiting just beyond the effort you put in.

Chapter V.

Cultivating Lasting Fulfillment

A. Identifying Individual Happiness and Fulfillment

In order to cultivate lasting fulfillment in a relationship, it's vital that both partners identify and pursue their individual sources of happiness and fulfillment. This means having a clear understanding of what makes you happy, what your passions are, and what you need to feel fulfilled in life.

When each partner brings their own sense of happiness and fulfillment to the relationship, they are more likely to be happy together. Moreover, this encourages self-growth and independence. Each individual should have the space and support needed to pursue their interests and explore their passions without feeling guilty or inadequate.

B. Balancing Individual Needs with Partner's Needs

While it's important for partners to cultivate their own sense of happiness and fulfillment, it's also essential to balance these needs with the needs of the relationship. Being in a relationship entails a level of compromise and sacrifice for the greater good. This means finding a balance between individual needs and the needs of the relationship.

One way to do this is by identifying shared goals and values. By prioritizing these shared goals, partners can work together towards a common objective while still maintaining their individuality. Moreover, by acknowledging each other's needs and being willing to make compromises, couples create a sense of mutual respect and trust.

Another key component of balancing individual needs with the needs of the relationship is effective communication. Partners need to be able to communicate openly and honestly about their needs and desires. This includes being able to express dissatisfaction without fear of judgment or retaliation.

Overall, seeking fulfillment both individually and through the relationship requires a delicate balance. When partners can strike this balance, they create a roots of happiness, growth, and mutual support.

C. Embracing Change and Growth in Relationships

Change is an inevitable part of life, and relationships are no exception. It's important for couples to embrace the natural ebb and flow of their relationship and allow room for growth and evolution.

As individuals change and grow, so do their needs and desires. This means that a healthy relationship requires ongoing communication and flexibility to adapt to these changes. Partners need to be willing to support each other's personal growth and accommodate shifting priorities and interests.

Moreover, embracing change also means acknowledging that challenges and setbacks will inevitably arise. Couples who are able to approach difficult situations with kindness, compassion, and understanding are more likely to emerge from these challenges stronger and more connected than before.

Ultimately, cultivating lasting fulfillment in a relationship requires a willingness to embrace change and foster personal and relational growth. Partners should prioritize effective communication, mutual understanding, and the ability to adapt to changing circumstances. This may mean being willing to step out of their comfort zones and take risks in order to keep the relationship fresh and exciting.

Unlocking the Hidden Pillars of Intimacy

In addition, it's important to recognize that not all growth is positive. Relationships can experience setbacks, such as fights, misunderstandings, and other challenges. These experiences are an important part of fostering intimacy and promoting personal growth.

Rather than avoiding conflict, partners should work together to find positive ways to express their emotions and communicate their needs. Working through these difficult times together can lead to a deeper sense of understanding and connection.

In conclusion, cultivating lasting fulfillment in a relationship requires ongoing effort, dedication, and flexibility. By recognizing the importance of individual happiness, balancing individual needs with those of the relationship, and embracing change and growth, couples can create a deep and meaningful connection that stands the test of time. Through effective communication, mutual understanding, and a willingness to take risks and embrace change, couples can unlock the hidden pillars of intimacy and create something truly special.

Moreover, it's important to recognize that the journey towards fulfillment is not a destination. Relationships are an ongoing process, and require continuous attention, love, and care. So while it may not always be easy, couples who are willing to put in the effort can build a relationship that lasts a lifetime.

Finally, it's crucial to remember that each relationship is unique. What works for one couple may not work for another. It's important for each couple to find their own path towards fulfillment, and to do so with honesty, openness, and a deep commitment to each other.

Chapter VI.

Advanced Practices in Intimacy

A. Exploring Sensuality and Sexuality

Exploring sensuality and sexuality can be a powerful way to deepen intimacy in a relationship. This involves exploring both physical and emotional intimacy with your partner. Physical intimacy can include touch, kissing, and sex, while emotional intimacy involves sharing your innermost thoughts, feelings, and desires with your partner.

When it comes to exploring sensuality and sexuality, communication is key. Partners should feel comfortable expressing their needs and desires, as well as being able to honor and respect each other's boundaries. This can create a shared sense of trust that can deepen the sense of connection and intimacy between partners.

One way to explore sensuality and sexuality is through regular date nights. This can involve creating a romantic atmosphere, such as lighting candles or playing soft music, and engaging in activities that bring you both pleasure and joy. Reflecting on your partner's desires and needs can also be incredibly important. Additionally, exploring new ways of being intimate, such as experimenting with new positions or trying new techniques, can spice up the relationship and bring an element of excitement to the bedroom.

Exploring sensuality and sexuality can also involve taking the time to focus on self-care, such as mindfulness, meditation, and self-pleasure. By investing in your own pleasure and self-discovery, you can better connect with your own desires and communicate those effectively with your partner. It is about embracing your own sensuality, sexiness, and intrigue.

B. Managing Conflict and Challenges in Relationships

All relationships face challenges and conflicts at some point. Managing these challenges and conflicts effectively can be key to building deeper intimacy in a relationship. One important practice is to approach conflict with a mindset of curiosity and openness, rather than defensiveness or withdrawal.

It can also be helpful for couples to establish ground rules for how they will communicate during conflicts. For example, agreeing to avoid name-calling or yelling, and instead focusing on understanding the other person's perspective and needs.

Another advanced practice in managing conflict is learning to handle triggers. When disagreements arise, it's important for partners to become aware of their emotional triggers and how they react. This can involve mindfulness techniques such as deep breathing, or other stress-reducing exercises that help calm the mind and body.

Finally, one way to manage conflict in a relationship is to commit to a regular check-in process. This can involve setting aside time each week to discuss any issues that have arisen in the relationship and work together to find solutions. This can foster a sense of honesty and vulnerability between partners, as well as helping to maintain open lines of communication.

C. Honoring Self-Discovery and Development

Honoring self-discovery and development is another advanced practice that can deepen intimacy in a relationship. This means giving each partner space and support to pursue their individual interests, passions, and goals outside of the relationship.

Unlocking the Hidden Pillars of Intimacy

Encouraging each other's personal growth and development can have a positive impact on both partners and the relationship as a whole. It can create a sense of excitement, inspiration, and creativity, as well as a deeper appreciation for each other's unique qualities and capabilities.

Another aspect of self-discovery and development involves recognizing the importance of personal time and self-care. This can involve taking time to engage in hobbies, spending time with friends, or simply relaxing and unwinding by oneself. Prioritizing this time can help partners to feel more fulfilled, energized, and confident in themselves, which can then translate into a stronger relationship.

In order to honor self-discovery and development, couples may need to set boundaries and make compromises. This could involve taking turns supporting each other's interests, or agreeing on a regular schedule for personal time and activities. Additionally, it's important to recognize that personal growth and development can involve discomfort and sometimes failure. However, by embracing these challenges and encouraging each other to take risks, couples can deepen their connection and mutual understanding.

Overall, honoring self-discovery and development is about respecting each other's individuality and celebrating the unique qualities and talents that each partner brings to the relationship. By supporting personal growth and exploration, couples can create a foundation of trust, respect, and love that can lead to a deeply fulfilling and joyous partnership.

Chapter VII.

Intimacy in Different Areas of Life

A. Intimacy in Friendship and Familial Relationships

Intimacy isn't just limited to romantic relationships; it can also be cultivated in friendships and familial relationships. In fact, strong and meaningful connections with friends and family members can be just as rewarding as those found in romantic relationships.

To cultivate intimacy in these relationships, it's important to prioritize communication and vulnerability. This includes actively listening to loved ones, expressing empathy and support, and sharing one's own thoughts and feelings in an honest and open manner.

Cheryl Bach

Another way to deepen intimacy in friendship and familial relationships is by creating shared experiences and memories. This could involve traveling together, trying new activities, or simply spending quality time together. Additionally, it's important to be consistent in our efforts to maintain and strengthen these relationships. This means regularly checking in with loved ones, celebrating milestones and achievements together, and making time for each other even when life gets busy.

B. Intimacy in Professional Relationships

Intimacy in professional relationships can be more challenging to achieve, but it's just as important as intimacy in personal relationships. Building strong connections with colleagues and co-workers can lead to increased job satisfaction, better teamwork, and a more positive work environment.

Unlocking the Hidden Pillars of Intimacy

One way to cultivate intimacy in professional relationships is by practicing active listening and empathy. This means really hearing what others have to say, acknowledging their perspectives, and showing that we care about their thoughts and feelings.

Additionally, taking the time to get to know colleagues on a personal level can also help build intimacy in the workplace. This could involve talking about shared interests or hobbies, or even engaging in team building activities outside of work. Celebrating colleagues' achievements and milestones, showing appreciation, and offering support during difficult times can also help foster intimacy in professional relationships.

C. Intimacy in the Digital Age

The rise of technology and social media has opened up new avenues for intimacy in the digital age. However, it's important to balance our digital connections with real-life relationships and experiences.

One way to cultivate intimacy in the digital age is by being intentional about our online interactions. This means taking the time to really connect with others online and engage in meaningful conversations. It also involves being mindful of how our digital lives impact our mental health and well-being.

Another way to build intimacy in the digital age is by using technology to enhance our real-life relationships. This could involve keeping in touch with out-of-town friends and family members, or even using video chat to have face-to-face conversations with loved ones who live far away. Additionally, social media can be used as a tool to create and maintain relationships with people who share similar interests or experiences.

Unlocking the Hidden Pillars of Intimacy

However, it's important to be aware of the potential downsides of relying too heavily on digital connections. In some cases, social media and other online platforms can actually hinder intimate connections by promoting comparisons, feelings of inadequacy, and superficial interactions. Thus, it's important to use technology intentionally and mindfully, keeping in mind the importance of real-life connections.

In conclusion, intimacy can be cultivated in a variety of settings and relationships, from personal partnerships to friendships, familial relationships, and even professional connections. By prioritizing communication, vulnerability, shared experiences, and intentional connections, we can build deeper and more meaningful connections that enrich our lives in countless ways. Whether through face-to-face conversations, meaningful online interactions, or a combination of both, intimacy is a vital component of our overall well-being and happiness. By recognizing and honoring the hidden pillars of intimacy, we can unlock the potential for deep emotional bonds, authentic relationships, and lasting fulfillment in love, life, and beyond.

Chapter VIII.

Conclusion

A. Key Takeaways

Throughout this book, we've explored the many facets of intimacy and how they can be used to build deep emotional bonds, nurture authentic relationships, and cultivate lasting fulfillment in love, life, and beyond.

From the importance of vulnerability and communication to the power of shared experiences and intentional connections, we've uncovered a wealth of insights and strategies for unlocking the hidden pillars of intimacy in our lives.

One of the key takeaways from this book is that intimacy is a vital component of human connection and plays a powerful role in creating a fulfilling life. Whether we're cultivating intimacy in romantic relationships, friendships, familial relationships, or professional connections, the benefits of deepening our connections are far-reaching and cross-cutting.

We've also learned about the different types of intimacy, including physical, emotional, and intellectual intimacy, and how each of these contributes to building strong and meaningful connections with others. Moreover, we've explored the challenges that come with cultivating intimacy in various settings, from navigating conflict to balancing digital connections with real-life relationships.

B. Encouragement to Apply Lessons in Life

While this book has provided us with an abundance of knowledge and insights into the different ways we can cultivate intimacy in our lives, the real power is in applying these lessons to our own lives. This requires intentionality, vulnerability, and an openness to new experiences and connections.

It's important to remember that building intimacy is a process that takes time and effort, and there will undoubtedly be obstacles along the way. However, by committing to practicing the strategies and insights outlined in this book, we can move closer towards living a more fulfilling life filled with deep and authentic connections.

Remember that cultivating intimacy is not a one-size-fits-all process. Each person and relationship is unique, and it's essential to allow space for personal growth and exploration. As we continue on our journey towards deeper connections, it's okay to stumble and make mistakes. These challenges provide learning opportunities for us to grow individuals and as partners or friends.

C. The Power of Intimacy in Creating a Fulfilling Life

In conclusion, intimacy unlocks the power of human connection and plays a vital role in creating a fulfilling life. Whether we're connecting with others emotionally, physically, or intellectually, intimacy allows us to build deep, meaningful, and lasting relationships that bring us joy, purpose, and love.

Unlocking the hidden pillars of intimacy requires vulnerability, communication, intentionality, and shared experiences. It also requires a willingness to be open to personal growth and to embrace change and new connections.

The benefits of cultivating intimacy extend beyond just our personal lives. Intimacy also plays a potent role in professional relationships, helping us to foster teamwork, inspire innovation, and create a positive and supportive work culture.

By recognizing the importance of intimacy in all areas of our lives and committing to building deeper connections, we unlock the potential for a life that is abundant in love, joy, and fulfillment. We hope this book has provided you with the tools and insights you need to start your journey towards unlocking the hidden pillars of intimacy and creating a more fulfilling life.

Cheryl Bach